High-Alert Medications and Safe Practices

A study guide for nurses

MARLA HUSCH, RPh
JENNIFER M. GROSZEK, RN, BSN, MJ
DENISE ROONEY, RN, BSN, OCN

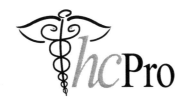

High-Alert Medications and Safe Practices: A study guide for nurses is published by HCPro, Inc.

HCPro, Inc., provides information resources for the healthcare industry.

HCPro, Inc., is not affiliated in any way with the Joint Commission on Accreditation of Healthcare Organizations, which owns the JCAHO trademark.

Marla Husch, RPh, Author
Jennifer M. Groszek, RN, BSN, MJ, Author
Denise Rooney, RN, BSN, OCN, Author
John Gettings, Managing Editor
Lauren Rubenzahl, Copy Editor
Jean St. Pierre, Creative Director
Jackie Diehl Singer, Graphic Artist
Michael Michaud, Layout Artist
Shane Katz, Cover Designer
Kathy Levesque, Group Publisher
Suzanne Perney, Publisher

Advice given is general. Readers should consult professional counsel for specific legal, ethical, or clinical questions.

Arrangements can be made for quantity discounts.

For more information, contact:
HCPro, Inc.
200 Hoods Lane
P.O. Box 1168
Marblehead, MA 01945
Telephone: 800/650-6787 or 781/639-1872
Fax: 781/639-2982
E-mail: *customerservice@hcpro.com*

Visit HCPro, Inc., at its World Wide Web sites:
www.hcpro.com and www.hcmarketplace.com

CONTENTS

ABOUT THE AUTHORS

Marla Husch, RPh

Marla Husch, RPh, has more than 10 years of clinical experience at a tertiary-care academic medical center. She has made significant contributions to academically rigorous and practically useful patient safety research.

After serving as a clinical pharmacist in both oncology and large organ transplant programs at Northwestern Memorial Hospital, she became a member of the institution's patient safety research team. Composed of dedicated nurses, pharmacists, and physicians, the team has generated research and publications of importance in the patient safety field and on patient care and operational improvements. It is an authority on patient safety measurement and improvement.

Husch earned her bachelor's degree at the Purdue University School of Pharmaceutical Sciences (West Lafayette, IN). She has been a member of several professional organizations during her career, including the American Society of Health-System Pharmacists, the Illinois Cancer Pain Initiative, and the American Society of Parenteral and Enteral Nutrition (ASPEN). She also serves as a course faculty member for the Department of Physical Therapy and Human Movement Sciences at the Northwestern University Feinberg School of Medicine.

Jennifer M. Groszek, RN, BSN, MJ

Jennifer Groszek, RN, BSN, MJ, has six years of healthcare experience in the acute-care setting. She has participated in a variety of process improvements, specifically medication safety initiatives and patient fall prevention.

She began her career as a registered nurse with the neurosurgery patient population. As a research nurse coordinator on Northwestern Memorial Hospital's patient safety research team, she participated in numerous quality initiatives and patient safety efforts by examining systems and errors, conducting surveillance activities via observation record review, assisting with data analysis, and providing education and consultation to clinicians.

Groszek earned her bachelor's degree in nursing from Saint Mary's College, Notre Dame, and her master of jurisprudence in health law from Loyola University's School of Law in Chicago.

Denise Rooney, RN, BSN, OCN

Denise Rooney, RN, BSN, OCN, has more than 17 years of experience in acute academic healthcare. She has a strong clinical background, with in-depth knowledge of oncology nursing, chemotherapeutics, and patient safety. Committed to personnel training and development, she has coordinated many nursing educational programs.

As patient safety is her area of focus, she manages a patient safety research and demonstration team at a large academic medical center in the Midwest. The team has generated research and publications in the areas of safety and quality and has initiated a host of critically important research related to patient care and operational improvements.

Rooney earned her bachelor's degree at Marquette University. She has worked at Northwestern Memorial Hospital and Northwestern University Medical School in operations, research, safety, and quality. She has been a member of the Oncology Nursing Society for the majority of her career and obtained Certification in 1990. Her professional memberships include the National Patient Safety Foundation, Patient Safety Officer Society, and the American Organization of Nurse Executives.

ACKNOWLEDGEMENTS

We thank the following reviewers for providing their time and expertise in reviewing the contents of this educational program and for their efforts to improve patient safety.

Cindy Barnard, MBA, MSJS, Director Quality Strategies

Anne Bobb, RPh, Patient Safety Team/Insulin Task Force

Bill Budris, RPh, Drug Information Center

Lisa Cieplechowicz, NM Academy

John Clarke, MD, Patient Safety and Geriatrics

Anthony DeSantis, MD, Endocrinology, Internal Medicine

Kari Foote, RN, Advanced Practice Nurse, Oncology

Mike Fotis, RPh, Pharmacy Manager

Kristine Gleason, RPh, Patient Safety Team

Travis Hunerdosse, RPh, Clinical Staff Pharmacist, Practice Coordinator

Tracie Jacobson, RPh, Anticoagulation Service

Misty Kirby-Nolan, RN, Advanced Practice Nurse, Pain

Desi Kotis, PharmD, Pharmacy Manager

Michele Langenfeld, Director, Surgical Nursing

Scott Lothian, RPh, Analgesic Dosing Service

Mary Majewski, RN, PCC, MICU

Debbie Mast, RN, Resource Coordinator Oncology

Joanna Maudlin, RPh, Anticoagulation Service

Vita Mikalunas, RN, Nutritional Support Team

Karen Nordstrom, Director of Pharmacy

Gary Noskin, MD, Medical Director, Infection Control and Prevention

Katie Opfer, RN, Clinical Quality

Judy Paice, RN, PhD, Director Cancer Pain Program

William Peruzzi, MD, Critical Care Medicine, Anesthesiology

Judith Reymond, NM Academy

Halina Rubin, RPh, Nutritional Support Team

Joy Springer, RN, Certified Diabetic Educator

Marilyn Szekendi, RN, Patient Safety Team

This educational program was supported by the state of Illinois Department of Public Aid and Northwestern Memorial Hospital and the U.S. Public Health Service grant UR8/515081 (Dr. Noskin).

Introduction

This book is designed to offer practical, immediate support to bedside nurses in American acute care hospitals. While the patient safety literature increasingly implicates a relatively small number of medications as the source of the most serious errors and instances of patient harm, there is a lack of tools available to improve the knowledge base of staff who care for patients every day.

Medications are the foundation of healthcare for untold millions of Americans every day: healing, ameliorating pain and symptoms, and sustaining life. Yet it is also estimated that medication errors cause 7,000 or more deaths per year in the United States as well as significant harm and injury from incorrect dosing, omissions, and other errors.

Current research shows that a majority of medication errors contributing to death or serious injury involve a small number of specific medications. The Institute for Safe Medication Practices and the Joint Commission on Accreditation of Healthcare Organizations have termed these "high-alert medications." Both organizations recommend focused attention on staff competence in administering these medications.

We also know that it is the administration phase of medication use that is most dangerous. Although studies vary, some of the most rigorous work suggests that more errors resulting in preventable adverse drug events occur during prescribing (56%) than during administration (34%) of medications. However, errors during administration are far more likely to reach the patient and cause harm. This study concluded that 48% of prescribing errors were detectable and none of the administration errors were caught.[1] Extensive and creative work is under way to engineer solutions to the problem of medication error at the point of administration. Technologies are being developed and used in some sites, employing bar coding to match the patient, medication, and order to prevent errors at the bedside. So-called "smart" infusion pumps are evolving with safety features ranging from crude dose limits to full integration with an electronic medical record, dose and order checking, and documentation.

Once matured, these technologies are likely to dominate the future of patient safety efforts and make the administration of medications safer. In the meantime, and even with the promise of future technologies, it is imperative that healthcare professionals be knowledgeable about the medications they prescribe and administer, and that they be provided with the very best orientation and education to equip them to protect their patients from inadvertent harm. That is the purpose of this book.

This text was developed and tested at a large, complex, academic medical center, and it has been enthusiastically received by our colleagues. We are all pleased to offer it to the wider community and hope that it will be as welcomed in your environment as it has in ours.

Marla Husch, RPh
Research Pharmacist, Patient Safety

Jennifer Groszek, RN, BSN, MJ
Risk Manager

Denise Rooney, RN, BSN, OCN
Manager, Patient Safety

Cynthia Barnard, MBA, CPHQ
Director, Quality Strategies

Reference

1. D.W. Bates, D. Cullen, N. Laird, et al. "Incidence of adverse drug events and potential adverse drug events: implications for prevention." *Journal of the American Medical Association.* 1995;274:29–34.

General safety principles

The following safety principles are applicable to the administration of all medications:

- Two unique patient identifiers should be assessed prior to administering medications. Reliable choices include those on the wristband or those that the patient can verbalize, such as name, age/date of birth, and medical record number. Never use room number or location as an identifier.
- Allergy status is assessed prior to administration.
- The nurse understands the medication's intended purpose and ensures the "Five Rights":

    1. Right patient
    2. Right dose
    3. Right route
    4. Right frequency
    5. Right time

- The nurse documents in a timely manner having checked the five rights.
- The patient is informed of the drug, dose, potential side effects, and any relevant laboratory values.
- "Read back and verify" is performed by anyone receiving a telephone or verbal order.
- Only hospital-approved abbreviations, acronyms, and symbols are used in documentation.
- Many medications have distinctive colors. However, never rely on color to identify a medication.
- Any medication error, near miss, or adverse drug reaction should be reported according to your institution's incident report system policy. You may also report systems (e.g., pumps, dispensing systems, human systems, etc.) that appear vulnerable to error so that they can be improved.
- Consult the pharmacy as a reference for questions.
- Syringes not prepared at the bedside are labeled with the name of the medication and dose.
- A double check system is often used with the administration of certain high-alert medications. Double checks require two clinicians to independently calculate the dose without reviewing prior calculations. This can ensure

    1. detection of error before it reaches a patient
    2. early identification of systems vulnerable to human error so that they can be improved[1]

Reference

1. *The road less traveled.* Huntingdon Valley, PA. Institute for Safe Medication Practices. 2002 August 21.

Opioids

Why are opioids identified as high-alert medications?

Opioids bind with opiate receptors at many sites in the central nervous system (e.g., brain, brain stem, spinal cord, etc.) and peripheral nervous system, and thereby alter both the perception of and emotional response to pain. If they are prescribed, administered, or monitored inappropriately, respiratory depression, coma, and even death can result.

As you read this section, keep in mind these commonly reported problems associated with opioids:

- Misconceptions about addiction, tolerance, dependence, and allergies.
- Misunderstandings regarding equianalgesic dosing of opioids.
- Infusion pump errors with Patient Controlled Analgesia (PCA) and Patient Controlled Epidural Analgesia (PCEA) are frequent.[1]
- Oral liquid versions of morphine and oxycodone are available in many concentrations. Mix-ups among them have led to serious overdoses.[2]
- Allergic reactions occur frequently.[3]
- Errors related to the drug, concentration, and route.
- Confusion between hydromorphone, morphine, and oxycodone:
  - Hydromorphone intravenous (IV) is five times more potent than morphine IV
  - Oral hydromorphone is about three times more potent than oxycodone
- Families and friends push the PCA or PCEA button, which can lead to serious overdoses.[4]
- Patients receiving opioids may not be adequately monitored. This is critical during the first 24 hours and at night because nocturnal hypoxia occurs most frequently during these periods.[5]
- Confusion has occurred between sustained-release and immediate-release products (e.g., Oxycontin and oxycodone).

Back pain

Below is a case study about a patient who was at risk for overdose because of inappropriate dosing and administration of morphine.

A 58-year-old man with chronic lower back pain is admitted to your unit with a PCA after a laminectomy. His PCA orders read "morphine 2 mg every eight minute bolus with no basal dose." He was taking Norco (one tablet every six hours) at home for several months prior to the surgery. He is complaining of severe pain, and you notice that his wife is pressing the button on the PCA. What is wrong with this picture?

Source: Northwestern Memorial Hospital Pain Expert Nurse Newsletter (November 2002).

- First, the bolus on a PCA should not be set at eight minutes. Remember that the peak effect of most intravenous opioids is 15 minutes, so boluses given more frequently can lead to accumulation of the drug and potential sedation. Eventually, such accumulation can lead to respiratory depression.

- Second, determine the patient's previous opioid dose. Norco, or 10 mg of hydrocodone, is approximately equal to 10 mg of oral morphine. The patient was taking four doses each day, or 40 mg, which is approximately equal to 40 mg of oral morphine or 13.3 mg of parenteral morphine. Thus, the best method of replacing his previous opioid dose would be to convert the 13 mg of parenteral morphine into a basal rate of approximately 0.5 mg per hour. Contact your pharmacy for assistance.

- Third, to determine whether the bolus dose is correct, ask the patient how much relief he obtains with the 2 mg. If the pain is relieved 100% and he is sedated, then reduce the bolus. If the pain is relieved 100% and he is not sedated, the dose is correct. And if the relief is less than 100%, even with the addition of the basal rate, then increase the bolus dose. Normally we use 50%–100% of the hourly rate, which would be 0.25 mg–0.5 mg. But this dose only replaces his previous Norco dose. Reassessment is critical to determine the effective dose.

- Fourth, educate the patient's wife about the dangers of anyone other than the patient pushing the button on the PCA pendant. Most family members or friends will be responsive. Consult the physician and consider a care conference if they continue to interfere.

Critical thinking

- Is the current regimen providing relief to the patient's satisfaction?
- Does the patient or the patient's family have misconceptions about opioid use? (e.g, fear of addiction, tolerance, dependence, etc.)[6]
- Does the patient have unrealistic expectations of pain control?
- Does a pharmacist need to be consulted?
- Are there any new complaints or physical assessment changes that may relate to the use of the pain medications?
- Is there an appropriate bowel regimen prescribed?
- Does the patient have undesirable past experiences with the use of opioids (e.g., effectiveness, adverse effects, history of substance abuse, etc.)?[7]
- Are there concomitant orders for medications that contain acetaminophen? (If so, monitor for total daily doses of acetaminophen.)
- If a PCA is ordered for a patient, is the patient a suitable candidate based on his or her level of consciousness, psychological reasons, or intellectual capacity?

Nursing implications

Administration

- Opioids may be administered through a variety of routes: oral, transdermal, rectal, and parental (which includes IV, subcutaneous (SQ), epidural, and intrathecal).
- Although some pain medications are prescribed to be administered intramuscularly, this method is not recommended because the absorption is highly variable. Contact the physician to determine alternative routes that may be available.[8]
- Prior to administration, assess baseline
    - pain level
    - sedation level
    - respiratory status
- Verify established opioid use prior to initiating an opioid regimen.
- Assess for treatment contraindications, such as concomitant opioids that have the same duration of action.
- Contact pharmacy regarding potential incompatibility concerns with IV analgesic medications.
- Assess the need for an appropriate bowel regimen to help prevent constipation.

- All opioids are not equianalgesic. For example, 2 mg IV hydromorphone is approximately equal to 10 mg IV morphine.
- Opioids, even at appropriate doses, can suppress respiration, heart rate, and blood pressure. Frequent monitoring is therefore essential.[9]

Monitoring

- Use a pain intensity scale to assess patient's response to treatment. (For further guidance, refer to Exhibit 1.1 on p. 12)
- Monitor "PRN" (as needed) use. Decreasing use may indicate decreasing pain, and orders may need to be adjusted.[10]
- Monitor
    - respiratory status
    - sedation level
    - nausea/vomiting
    - bowel/bladder function

(For additional guidance on monitoring and assessing respiratory status and sedation level, use the sample sedation scale and respiratory rate monitoring guidelines in Exhibit 1.2 on p. 13 for additional guidance.)

- Monitor total daily acetaminophen intake for patients taking combination opioid products (e.g., patients with normal liver function should not receive greater than 4000 mg/day.) (To review the aceteaminophen content of several common preparations, refer to Exhibit 1.3 on p. 14.)
- Dosing should be reevaluated if the cause or focus of the pain changes (e.g., postoperative, postprocedure, etc.) or is removed (e.g., tubes, renal stones, etc.).

Oral opioids

- Sustained-release oral medications cannot be crushed or split.
- When reviewing medication orders, be vigilant for similar trade and generic names. For example,

> Roxanol is morphine (immediate release, liquid)
> Roxicodone is oxycodone (immediate release)
> and
> MS Contin is morphine (long-acting)
> OxyContin is oxycodone (long-acting)

- Oral liquid opioids are available in various concentrations, which can be stored in proximity to each other. For example, Roxicodone is available in 5 mg/mL bottles or 20 mg/mL bottles.

- Be aware that potencies of IV and oral preparations are not equianalgesic. For example, 30 mg of oral morphine is approximately equal to 10 mg IV/SQ morphine.

- Note products that combine an opioid and acetaminophen (refer to Exhibit 1.2 on p. 13):
    - Norco contains hydrocodone 10 mg/acetaminophen 325 mg
    - Vicodin contains hydrocodone 5 mg/acetaminophen 500 mg

- Watch for concomitant orders for acetaminophen, such as
    - *Tylenol Extra Strength, 1–2 tablets po every 6 hours PRN*
    - *Norco, 1–2 tablets po every 4 hours PRN*

- The total daily dose of acetaminophen should not exceed 4000 mg in patients with normal liver function.

Transdermal opioids

- Remove old patches prior to placing new ones (when appropriate) on alternate sites (e.g., flat sites such as the back or chest are best).

- Treat topical patches like any other medication: chart on the Medication Administration Record when it was administered and on what site.[11]

- Medication from transdermal patches can be absorbed to a much greater extent in patients with elevated body temperatures (e.g., from a warming blanket or fever). This can lead to significant overdoses.[12]

PCA

- PCA infusions are always used in conjunction with a maintenance intravenous fluid.

- It is recommended that PCA cartridge concentrations be standard throughout an institution. For example, only 1 mg/mL and 0.2 mg/mL are available for use. It is also recommended that colored labels differentiate these concentrations. However, do not rely only on color to differentiate.

- The button should never be pushed by anyone else, including friends or family members.[13]

- Educate patients about the proper use of PCA before initiation. Start during the preoperative testing visit so that patients are not too groggy to understand.[14]

- PCA tubing should be changed if there is a medication change or concentration change.

- The pump history should be cleared only if there is a medication change, such as morphine to hydromorphone. If there is only a concentration change, such as hydromorphone 0.2 mg/mL to hydromorphone 1 mg/mL, the history should not be cleared.

- It is recommended that two registered nurses check and verify the PCA pump settings at time of initiation and/or change in dose, medication, concentration, or medication cartridge.

- Research shows that double checks are most effective when conducted independently.[15]

PCEA

- PCEA is contraindicated in patients receiving low molecular weight heparin or fibrinolytic therapy.
- No other medications should be infused through the epidural line.
- If a bolus dose is administered through the epidural catheter, the nurse should stay at the bedside during and for five minutes following administration of the bolus dose.
- To avoid overdosing, the maximum bolus volume should not exceed the current hourly rate of infusion.
- The epidural catheter may be left in place after discontinuing the infusion. A lock is placed at the distal end of the catheter and does not need to be flushed. The epidural space is free space and is not prone to clotting.
- It is recommended that two registered nurses check and verify the PCEA pump settings at the time of initiation and/or change in dose, medication, concentration, or medication cartridge.
- Research shows that double checks are most effective when conducted independently.[16]

IV opioids

- Verify the concentration on the pharmacy label.
- Calculate the continuous infusion rate and independently check with another nurse or pharmacist.
- Never use a continuous infusion rate for acute pain of a limited duration.[17]
- When assessing the need for a possible change in the hourly continuous infusion rate, consider the total usage (including number of bolus doses used) over at least the previous 12 hours. If only the first few hours are considered, the need for an increase in the hourly rate may appear falsely elevated as many times more boluses are required at the initiation of pain control medication until steady-state is achieved.
- To prevent overdosing, bolus doses are preferred to increases in the hourly continuous infusion rate to treat episodic or sporadic pain.[18]

Exercise

Your patient's current pain medication orders are as follows:

Tylenol Extra Strength 1–2 tablets po every 6 hours PRN and Norco 1–2 tablets po every 4 hours PRN

It is 2100 and the patient has already received two tablets of Tylenol Extra Strength at 0100, 0700, and 1600 that day. He also has received Norco (two tablets at 1200 after physical therapy). The patient is now requesting two more tablets of Norco before he goes to sleep. What should you do?

Answer provided on p. 57.

Summary points

- Errors associated with opioids are among the most commonly reported incidents that lead to patient harm. Overdoses have occurred due to
    - confusion between different opioids because of sound-alike names.
    - anyone other than the patient pushing the button on the PCA or PCEA.
    - the fact that even at appropriate doses, opioids can suppress respiration, heart rate, and blood pressure. Frequent monitoring is therefore essential.
    - failure to monitor total daily amounts of acetaminophen intake, which can lead to severe liver damage.
- Independent double checks are recommended for rate calculations and infusion pump programming so that errors can be identified prior to administration.

Exhibit 1.1 | **Patient pain-assessment tool**

- It is important to let your doctors and nurses know when you are in pain.
- Point to where the pain is located.
- Describe how the pain feels (e.g., aching, throbbing, or burning). There may be many ways to describe your pain.
- Rate your pain on a scale of 0–10, with 0 meaning no pain and 10 meaning the worst pain you could imagine.

Wong-Baker FACES pain rating scale

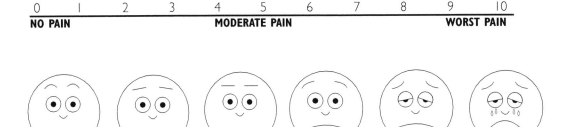

| 0 | 1 | 2 | 3 | 4 | 5 | 6 | 7 | 8 | 9 | 10 |
| NO PAIN | | | | MODERATE PAIN | | | | | WORST PAIN | |

Source: Wong D.L., Hockenberry-Eaton M., Wilson D., Winkelstein M.L., Schwarz P.: Wong's Essentials of Pediatric Nursing ed. 6, St. Louis, 2001, p. 1301. Copyright Mosby, Inc. Reprinted with permission.

Exhibit 1.2 | **Sedation scale and respiratory rate monitoring guidelines**

Patient-controlled analgesia (PCA)	Epidural and patient-controlled epidural analgesia (PCEA)
Sedation scale and respiratory rate: every two hours for 24 hours, then every four hours thereafter.	Sedation scale and respiratory rate: every two hours for 24 hours, then every four hours thereafter. Same monitoring frequency following initiation of epidural infusion, after a bolus, and/or increase in rate.

Sedation scale

S   Sleeping   Normal sleep, respiration rate > 8 per minute
0   None   Alert, awake
1   Mild   Responds to normal voice
2   Moderate   Responds to loud voice/shaking
3   Severe   Somnolent, difficult to arouse

Sensory motor checks

If *bupivacaine* is used, check lower extremities every two hours, while awake, for the first 24 hours.

0   Normal strength and sensation
1   Weak but able to bend knees and ankles, normal sedation
2   Unable to bend knees, normal sensation
3   Unable to move legs, decreased sensation

  • Monitor blood pressure every hour for four hours, then every four hours thereafter
  • Check orthostatic blood pressure prior to ambulating

Exhibit 1.3 — Acetaminophen hepatoxicity

It is necessary to monitor the total acetaminophen intake for patients taking combination opioid products. The oral adult analgesic dose of acetaminophen is 325 mg–1000 mg. The total daily dose should not exceed 4000 mg. Recognition of the quantities of acetaminophen provided by various combination analgesic products can help to prevent unintended ingestion of potentially toxic doses. The following table details the acetaminophen content of several common preparations.

TRADE NAME	ACETAMINOPHEN CONTENT	OPIOID	NUMBER OF TABLETS/CAPSULES TO REACH 4 G/DAY
Vicodin®	500 mg	Hydrocodone 5 mg	8
Vicodin Extra Strength®[1]	750 mg	Hydrocodone 7.5 mg	5
Darvocet N-100®[1]	650 mg	Propoxyphene 100 mg	6
Norco®	325 mg	Hydrocodone 10 mg	12
Tylenol®	325 mg	Not applicable	12
Tylenol Extra Strength®	500 mg	Not applicable	8
Tylenol #3®	300 mg	Codeine 30mg	13
Tylenol #4®	300 mg	Codeine 60 mg	13
Percocet-5/325®	325 mg	Codeine 5 mg	12

[1]Although effective for many types of moderate to severe pain, combination agents have a maximum or ceiling dose due to the acetaminophen. Thus, Vicodin Extra Strength® and Darvocet N-100® are not recommended, as their acetaminophen content is high.

It is best to use only one of these agents at a time. When these agents are prescribed at close to the maximum acetaminophen dose, it is necessary to inform patients not to use acetaminophen containing over-the-counter (OTC) analgesics, sinus/allergy medicine, or cough-cold remedies.

Source: Reprinted with permission from Michael Fotis, M.A. (Ed). Optimizing medication use at NMH: Suggested guidelines for commonly encountered problems. Chicago: Northwestern Memorial Hospital, 2003.

References

1. M.R. Cohen and C.M. Kilo. "High-alert medications: Safeguarding against errors." In M.R. Cohen (Ed.), *Medication Errors*. Washington, DC: American Pharmaceutical Association, 1999.
2. Ibid.
3. Ibid.
4. Ibid.
5. "Safety issues with patient-controlled analgesia." Huntingdon Valley, PA: Institute for Safe Medication Practices (ISMP), 2003 July 10.
6. M. Fotis, M.A. (Ed.) Optimizing medication use at NMH: Suggested guidelines for commonly encountered problems. Chicago: Northwestern Memorial Hospital, 2003.
7. Ibid.
8. J. Paice. "Alternative to intramuscular pain medication." Northwestern Memorial Hospital *Pain Expert Nurse Newsletter*. 2003 January.
9. "More on avoiding opiate toxicity." Huntingdon Valley, PA: ISMP, 2002 May 29.
10. See note 6 above.
11. "Serious consequences if patches are not removed." Huntingdon Valley, PA: ISMP, 2003 June 26.
12. "Elevated skin and body temperatures." Huntingdon Valley, PA: ISMP, 2003 June 30.
13. "Safety issues with patient-controlled analgesia." Huntingdon Valley, PA: ISMP, 2003 July 10.
14. See note 8 above.
15. "Maybe Santa's on to something." Huntingdon Valley, PA: ISMP, 2001 December 12.
16. Ibid.
17. See note 6 above.

Intravenous heparin

Why is heparin identified as a high-alert medication?

Unfractionated heparin is a parenteral anticoagulant widely used in clinical practice. It accelerates the activity of antithrombin III to inactivate thrombin. Serious, even fatal bleeding (if supratherapeutic) and thrombotic events (if subtherapeutic) can occur if it is dosed, administered, or monitored inappropriately.

As you read this section, keep in mind these commonly reported problems associated with heparin:

- Calculation and dosing errors are frequent.[1]
- Heparin is commonly confused with other medications. For example, the Institute for Safe Medication Practice reports that insulin and heparin vials may be mistaken for one another because both are dosed in units, come in vials that look similar, and are sometimes stored in close proximity to each other.[2]
- Programming a heparin bolus rate on a pump and forgetting to reset the pump to the continuous infusion rate can lead to serious errors.[3]
- When prescribing heparin, if "units" is not spelled out, the u can be mistaken for a zero and lead to a 10-fold overdose.[4]
- When "cc" is used as an abbreviation for mL, the c's have been mistaken for zeros, leading to overdose.
- Infusion pump programming errors have led to serious and fatal events.
- Monitoring to measure the intensity of anticoagulation can be inconsistent (e.g., activated Partial Thromboplastin Time (aPTT) ordered or drawn at inappropriate frequency, time, or site).

Case study

A patient was receiving 1100 units/hour of heparin continuously for the treatment of venous thromboembolism. After six hours of continuous infusion heparin, the aPTT was greater than 130. The dose was reduced, but the next aPTT was ordered to be drawn 24 hours later, instead of repeated in four to six hours. As a result, this patient experienced unanticipated serious bleeding.

This is an example of the serious consequences that can occur if heparin is not appropriately monitored.

Critical thinking

- Was the weight in kilograms (kg) used for dosing?
- Was the aPTT both appropriately ordered and at the correct frequency when starting heparin or after dose changes?
- Does the reported lab value make sense?
- Does the calculated hourly infusion rate make sense?
- Does the patient have an underlying condition in which the clotting cascade is affected and may require closer monitoring (e.g., idiosyncratic thrombocytopenia)?
- Is the patient receiving any medications that might alter the anticoagulant effects of heparin?
- Were all concomitant heparin products such as enoxaparin or dalteparin discontinued prior to initiating heparin therapy?

Nursing implications

Administration

- Evaluate the order for correct dose and laboratory orders. (Remember that heparin is dosed per weight in kg.)
- Only administer intravenously via an infusion pump. (Please refer to Exhibit 2.1 on p. 21 for guidance on programming the infusion pump.)
- Heparin can be administered either intravenously (IV) or subcutaneously. Intramuscular (IM) injections can produce large hematomas if they accidentally puncture an IM vein.
- Independent double checks are recommended for rate calculations and infusion pump programming so that errors can be identified prior to administration.
- Prior to initiating heparin therapy, verify that the patient is not receiving concomitant heparin products such as enoxaparin or dalteparin.
- If a bolus is ordered, administer it from a vial obtained from the pharmacy. Do not modify the rate of the infusion.
- It is recommended that the concentrations of heparin infusions are standard throughout an entire institution to prevent rate calculation errors.

Monitoring

- The aPTT is used to measure the intensity of anticoagulation.[5]
- The target aPTT is 65–105 seconds.
- The aPTT is usually drawn four to six hours after initial dose or dose change.
- Communicate with the physician regarding concerns related to dose, rate, and appropriate lab monitoring.
- Monitor platelets to assess for heparin-induced thrombocytopenia.
- Indications for contacting the physician are
  1. gross hematuria
  2. hematoma formation
  3. incision or IV site with excessive bleeding or oozing
  4. platelets less than $100,000/mm^3$ or a decrease of $50,000/mm^3$
  5. hemoglobin decrease of more than two grams per deciliter (g/dL) or a total hemoglobin of less than 8g/dL.[6]
- Monitor for physical signs/symptoms of bleeding. Hemorrhagic complications may be manifested by signs or symptoms that do not indicate obvious bleeding.

Signs and symptoms that may indicate bleeding that is not otherwise obvious:

- Decreased blood pressure
- Decreased urine output
- Mental status changes
- Shortness of breath
- Pain in chest or abdomen
- Dizziness
- Decrease in hemoglobin and hematocrit
- Weakness
- Headache

Obvious signs of bleeding:

- Petechiae/excessive bruising
- Bleeding from gums
- Hematuria
- Coffee ground emesis
- Dark, tarry stools
- Nosebleed

Exercise

Order: *heparin continuous infusion at 1300 units/hour and a 5000 unit IV bolus.*

Determine how you would administer the bolus and calculate the rate of the continuous infusion.
The standard concentration for IV heparin is 25,000 units in a 250 mL bag. The concentration is equivalent to 100 units/mL.

Answer provided on p. 57.

Summary points

- Serious bleeding can result from inappropriate use of heparin. Accurate prescribing, administration, and monitoring is vital.
- Dosing is weight-based (in kg). Therefore, a recent and accurate weight is necessary.
- Concomitant heparin products, such as enoxaparin or dalteparin, are contraindicated.
- Independent double checks are recommended for rate calculations and infusion pump programming.
- Maintaining an appropriate laboratory monitoring regimen and communication of results is essential.
- Monitor for physical signs and symptoms of bleeding. Hemorrhagic complications may be manifested by signs and symptoms that do not indicate obvious bleeding.

Exhibit 2.1 — IV heparin administration

Administration of IV heparin is widely used for anticoagulation. Errors in dose, calculation, and infusion pump programming are common.

It is recommended that only one concentration of heparin for continuous infusion be available throughout an institution. The chart below is intended to serve as a reference to check before administering and programming the infusion pump. It is based on a standard concentration of 100 units/mL.

Remember, heparin dosing is based on weight in kg.

ADMINISTER: X UNITS/HOUR	RATE CALCULATION: X ML/HOUR
100	1
200	2
300	3
400	4
500	5
600	6
700	7
800	8
900	9
1000	10
1100	11
1200	12
1300	13
1400	14
1500	15
1600	16
1700	17
1800	18
1900	19
2000	20

For example, start a heparin continuous infusion at 1300 units/hour. What is the rate?

The calculation: $\dfrac{25,000 \text{ units}}{250 \text{ mL}} \quad \times \quad \dfrac{1300 \text{ units}}{x \text{ mL}}$

Answer: $100x = 1300$

Rate: $= 13 \text{mL/hour}$

If a bolus is ordered, obtain a vial from the pharmacy and administer it from a syringe rather than modifying the rate of the infusion (Regional Medical Safety Program for Hospitals, 2001).

Source: Regional Medical Safety Program for Hospitals, 2001, Northwestern Memorial Hospital. Reprinted with permission.

References

1. M.R. Cohen and C.M. Kilo. "High-alert medications: Safeguarding against errors." In M.R. Cohen (Ed.), *Medication Errors.* Washington, DC: American Pharmaceutical Association, 1999.

2. Ibid.

3. Ibid.

4. Ibid.

5. M. Fotis, M.A. (Ed.) *Optimizing medication use at NMH: Suggested guidelines for commonly encountered problems.* Chicago: Northwestern Memorial Hospital, 1999.

6. J. Hirsh, J.F. Dalen, D.R. Anderson, L. Poller, H. Bussey, J. Ansell, and D. Deykin. "Oral anticoagulants: Mechanism, action, clinical effectiveness and optimal therapeutic range." *Chest,* 119, 8S-21S, 2001.

Insulin

Why is insulin identified as a high-alert medication?

Insulin is a pancreatic hormone secreted by the beta-cells of the islets of Langerhans. It is essential for the metabolism of glucose and for the homeostasis of blood glucose. If it is dosed, administered, or monitored inappropriately, cardiac changes, electrolyte disturbances, seizures, coma, and even death can occur.

As you read this section, keep in mind the commonly reported problems associated with insulin:

- Fatalities have occurred when insulin is given in excessive amounts.[1]
- Clinicians have inadvertently confused heparin and insulin vials because both are similar in appearance, dosed in units, and often floor-stocked near one another.[2]
- When prescribing insulin, if "units" is not spelled out, the u can be mistaken for a zero and lead to a 10-fold overdose.[3]
- When "cc" is used as an abbreviation for mL, the c's have been mistaken for zeros, leading to overdose.
- Failure to recognize signs and symptoms of hyperglycemia/hypoglycemia.
- Long delays in insulin administration once a high blood glucose is obtained.[4]
- Confusion frequently arises due to similar names (e.g., Humalog and Humulin) and the many available strengths and concentrations.[5]
- Infusion pump programming errors associated with continuous infusions can be lethal because the onset of action for intravenous regular insulin is within 15 minutes, and the maximal effects occur within 15–30 minutes.
- Due to the wide variety of onset of actions for different insulins, administration in relationship to meals is complex.[6]
- Patients often require a regimen that includes more than one kind of insulin to manage their glucose levels. This adds to the complexity of insulin administration.[7]
- Insulin requirements vary and are dependent on multiple factors, including the type of diabetes, patient weight, concomitant medications, and changes in dietary intake.
- It's not uncommon for the onset of action, duration of action, and peak of onset to vary considerably between patients when the same type and amount of insulin is given.

Case study

A hospitalized patient is receiving a combination of insulin therapy: Lantus for basal-glucose control and Humalog as short-acting insulin. The patient was intended to receive 80 units of Lantus at bedtime. When the night nurse checked on her shortly after the start of the shift, the patient was unresponsive and her blood glucose level was 17. A quick investigation identified that the patient had received the bedtime dose of insulin using Humalog instead of Lantus.

Source: "Proliferation of insulin combination products," 2002.

This is an example of how mix-ups occur due to similar names and the variety of available strengths and concentrations.

Critical thinking

- Is the patient at increased risk for inadequate blood-glucose control due to underlying conditions, type of diabetes (e.g., Type 1 Diabetes Mellitus or Type 2 Diabetes Mellitus), food/medication interactions, medical management (i.e., nothing by mouth [NPO]), total parenteral nutrition, or steroids that are part of the current drug regimen?
- Is the patient at risk for hypokalemia (i.e., insulin drives potassium intracellularly)?
- Is the patient at risk for the development of diabetic ketoacidosis?
- Are the appropriate labs ordered to effectively monitor a patient who is receiving insulin and/or has been diagnosed with diabetes mellitus?
- Are the necessary labs drawn within an appropriate time interval in relation to administered doses?
- Are insulin doses administered within an appropriate time frame in relationship to meals?
- Was the patient informed of the insulin's name, dose, and glucose level before administration?
- Prior to discharge, did the patient receive education about insulin? It should include the importance of monitoring glucose levels, appropriate injection techniques, food/drug interactions, and prevention and management of hyperglycemia and hypoglycemia.

Nursing implications

Administration

- Obtain an accurate history of insulin therapy from patients.
- A variety of insulin preparations are available, many of which have different times of onset and duration. (Refer to Exhibit 3.1 on p. 27 for more administration guidance for some common insulin preparations.)
- Only regular insulin can be given intravenously, and it must be diluted in a solution, such as 0.9% sodium chloride.[8]
- Prior to discontinuing an insulin infusion, administer first dose of subcutaneous insulin as ordered. Continue administering the infusion for 30–60 minutes. This prevents rebound hyperglycemia.
- Tuberculin syringes should not be used to administer insulin. Only use insulin syringes. The metric scale may be confused with the apothecary scale on disposable syringes.[9]
- Inform the patient that he or she is receiving insulin. If insulin is not part of the medication regimen, the patient will often alert you to this and can prevent you from administering insulin to the wrong patient.[10]
- Educate your patient on signs, symptoms, and management of hyperglycemia and hypoglycemia.
- Independent double checks are recommended to gauge the insulin vial and withdrawn subcutaneous dose.
- Independent double checks are recommended for rate calculations and infusion pump programming so that errors can be identified prior to administration.
- If your patient is made NPO for a test or the tube feeds or total parenteral nutrition is stopped, address any changes in insulin needs.
- When a patient is receiving an intravenous (IV) insulin infusion, a separate line should be used for other IV medications and fluids.
- Each patient has his or her own insulin vial, which should be stored in the patient's individual medication drawer.

Monitoring

- If the patient requires hourly serum glucose monitoring, he or she should not leave the patient care area unattended.
- Communicate with the physician regarding desired blood-glucose parameters and goal values.
- Communicate with the physician regarding changes in dietary intake.
- Check the blood-glucose level after one hour following discontinuation of the insulin infusion. Then, if the patient is eating, check blood glucose levels before meals and at bedtime.
- Monitor for physical signs and symptoms of hyperglycemia/hypoglycemia. If either is suspected, check blood-glucose levels.

Signs and symptoms of hypoglycemia

- **Early**—hunger; weakness; shakiness; nervousness or anxiety; tachycardia; diaphoresis; tingling of lips, tongue, or fingers; pallor around the nose or mouth
- **Late**—dizziness, drowsiness, headache, inability to concentrate, crying, confusion, extreme fatigue, slurred speech, irritability, blurred or double vision, seizures, lack of coordination, coma

Signs and symptoms of hyperglycemia

- Polyuria, polyphagia, weakness, fatigue, blurred vision, dry mucous membranes, tachycardia, hypotension, polydipsia, glucosuria, poor skin turgor, confusion, tachypnea

Exercise

True or false: A general rule of thumb is that "clear" insulin is okay to be given intravenously.

Answer provided on p. 57.

Summary points

- Based on errors reported in literature, it is clear that serious harm can result from inappropriate management of insulin.
- Evaluation of the current glucose level prior to any insulin administration is critical to prevent life-threatening hypoglycemic episodes.
- Clinicians have inadvertently confused heparin and insulin vials because the vials look similar. Both are dosed in units, and both are floor-stocked items that are often stored near one another.
- Due to similar sounding names (e.g., Humalog and Humulin) and the multiple types and concentrations available, mix-ups can easily occur.
- Independent double checks are recommended for rate calculations and infusion pump programming when administering intravenous insulin infusions.
- Independent double checks are recommended to check the insulin vial and withdrawn subcutaneous dose.
- Inform a patient that he or she is receiving insulin. If insulin is not part of the medication regimen, the patient will often alert you to this and can prevent you from administering insulin to the wrong patient.

Exhibit 3.1 **Insulin preparations**

This table provides general information and is not intended to apply to every patient and situation. Individual response to insulin varies and is affected by temperature, site of injection, dose, physical activity, concomitant drug therapy, and other factors. Daily insulin doses, time of administration, diet, and exercise must be individualized and require continuous medical supervision. This table may not include all available brands of insulin.

	Insulin preparation	Onset (S)Q	Peak (h)	Duration (h)	Route	Time of administration
Rapid-acting	Insulin Lispro *Humalog*	0.25	0.5–1.5	3–5	Subcutaneous (SQ), SQ pump	Within 15 minutes before or immediately after a meal
Rapid-acting	Insulin Aspart *NovoLog*	0.25	1–3	3–5	SQ, SQ pump	Immediately (5–10 minutes) before meals
Rapid-acting	Insulin Regular Intravenous *Humulin R* *Novolin R*	0.25	0.25–0.5	0.5–1	IV	N/A
Short-acting	Insulin Regular *Humulin R* *Novolin R*	0.5–1	1–5	4–12	SQ, SQ pump	30–60 minutes before a meal
Intermediate-acting	Isophane Insulin Suspension *Humulin N* *Novolin N*	1–2	6–14	Up to 24	SQ only	Usually given 30–60 minutes before a meal or at bedtime
Intermediate-acting	Insulin Zinc Suspension (Lente) *Humulin L* *Novolin L*	1–3	6–14	16 to 24+	SQ only	Usually given 30–60 minutes before a meal or at bedtime
Long-acting	Insulin Glargine *Lantus*	1.1	No pronounced peak	Up to 24+	SQ only	Once daily at bedtime
Long-acting	Extended Insulin Zinc Suspension (Ultralente) *Humulin U*	4–8	8–20	Up to 28	SQ only	Usually given 30–60 minutes before a meal or at bedtime
Insulin combinations	Isophane Insulin Suspension and Regular Insulin *Humulin 70/30* *Humulin 50/50* *Novolin 70/30*	0.5	2–12	Up to 24	SQ only	30 minutes before a meal
Insulin combinations	Insulin Lispro Protamine Suspension and Insulin Lispro *Humalog Mix 75/25*	0.25	0.5–1.5	Up to 24	SQ only	Within 15 minutes of a meal
Insulin combinations	Insulin Aspart Protamine Suspension and Insulin Aspart *NovoLog Mix 70/30*	0.25	1–4	Up to 24	SQ only	10–20 minutes before a meal

Source: Reprinted with permission from K. Engelmann, Pharm.D, and M. Fotis, M.A. (Ed.) Optimizing medication use at NMH: Suggested guidelines for commonly encountered problems. Chicago: Northwestern Memorial Hospital, 2003.

References

1. M.R. Cohen and C.M. Kilo. "High-alert medications: Safeguarding against errors." In M.R. Cohen (Ed.), *Medication Errors*. Washington, DC: American Pharmaceutical Association, 1999.

2. Ibid.

3. Ibid.

4. J.M. Heatlie. "Reducing insulin medication errors evaluation of a quality improvement initiative." *Journal for Nurses in Staff Development,* 19, pp. 92–98, 2003.

5. See note 1 above.

6. "Complexity of insulin therapy." Huntingdon Valley, PA: Institute for Safe Medication Practices, 2003 April 17.

7. Ibid.

8. Ibid.

9. See note 1 above.

10. See note 1 above.

Electrolytes

Why are electrolytes (e.g., potassium chloride, sodium chloride 3% (hypertonic saline), magnesium, phosphorus, intravenous calcium) identified as high-alert medications?

Electrolytes are necessary components in the human body for the maintenance of nervous, muscular, and skeletal systems. If prescribed, administered, or monitored inappropriately, electrolyte abnormalities can lead to renal dysfunction or failure, cardiac arrest, coma, respiratory arrest, seizures, rhabdomyolysis (an acute, sometimes fatal disease characterized by destruction of the skeletal muscle), or death.

As you read this section, be aware of the commonly reported problems associated with electrolytes:

- Prescribers are often unaware of interactions that occur between calcium and phosphorus. Calcium phosphate may precipitate into the vasculature, resulting in organ injury.[1]
- Prescribers fail to indicate the desired salt when prescribing calcium. There is a three-fold difference in calcium amounts between calcium gluconate and calcium chloride.[2]
- Failure to consider that decreased albumin levels can make calcium serum levels appear falsely low when prescribing calcium supplementation.
- Potassium chloride has accidentally been given intravenous (IV) push, resulting in numerous fatalities.
- Use of long acting potassium products (such as K-Dur tablets) to correct severe hypokalemia rather than using an immediately absorbed product (such as K-Lor powder).
- The abbreviations for morphine sulfate (MSO_4) and magnesium sulfate ($MgSO_4$) have been mistaken for one another.[3]
- Confusion between "mg" (milligram) and "mEq" (millequivalent) has also led to serious errors.[4]
- Magnesium in concentrations of 25 g (Grams)/250 mL Normal Saline (NS) is only used to treat preeclampsia. This has been mistaken for 2 g/250 mL NS, which is indicated for electrolyte replacement.
- Confusion over appropriate routes of administration (e.g., calcium should never be given intramuscularly (IM) and concentrated potassium riders must be administered through a central line).
- Phosphorus preparations (both IV and oral) are only available in combination with sodium or potassium. Prescribers frequently fail to specify which salt is desired, and a patient who is at risk for hyperkalemia can inadvertently receive extra potassium.
- Some oral phosphorus supplements contain variable amounts of potassium. Due to confusion between products, hyperkalemia has occurred when treating hypophosphatemia.

- Intravenous calcium is frequently ordered in terms of "amps" or "vials" rather than exact dosage (e.g., "mEq").
- Infusion pump programming errors have led to patient harm.
- When a lab value is significantly different than a previous value, a lab error or blood draw error should be considered as a possibility when evaluating a change in therapy.

Case study

A bone marrow transplant patient had been receiving phosphorus replacement with two tablets TID of K Phos Neutral (8 millimoles (mMol) phosphorus, 1.1 mEq potassium and 13 mEq sodium). However, upon discharge, this was substituted with Neutra Phos K packets (8 mMol phosphorus, 14.25 mEq of potassium). The patient was hospitalized with hyperkalemia and electrocardiogram (EKG) abnormalities.

Source: "Look-alike/sound-alike drug names and other product-related issues." Huntingdon Valley, PA: Institute for Safe Medication Practice, 2002 April 3. Reprinted with permission.

This case study is an example of a commonly reported problem in which confusion between products due to sound-alike names can lead to a medication error with severe consequences.

Critical thinking

- Is the patient receiving any medications that may alter electrolyte levels (e.g., furosemide is a potassium-wasting diuretic; angiotensin-converting enzyme inhibitors, such as lisinopril promote potassium (K+) retention; oral quinolones, such as levofloxacin, bind to oral magnesium and calcium when administered concomitantly)?
- Is there a need to recheck a level? If so, when?
- Is the level consistent with the patient's clinical state?
- Is the patient receiving multiple concomitant electrolyte supplementation (e.g., the patient is receiving intravenous Dextrose 5% Water + 20 mEq of potassium chloride continuously for hydration prior to initiating chemotherapy; subsequently, a 60 mEq potassium chloride rider is ordered)?
- Is the intravenous route prescribed for a patient who could tolerate oral doses?
- Does the patient have cardiac instability? Should a transfer to a monitored setting be considered prior to IV electrolyte supplementation?

Nursing implications

General administration and monitoring considerations

- Check the patient's most recent electrolyte level prior to administration.
- Consider the dose of the supplement, both parenteral and oral, because it may need to be divided and administered in intervals.
- Evaluate renal function and replace cautiously in patients with renal impairment.
- Evaluate the most appropriate route of administration and duration of infusion.
- If a lab value is significantly different than a previous value, discuss with the physician the option of rechecking the level before changing the therapy.

Potassium chloride

Signs and symptoms of hypokalemia

Mild (symptoms usually absent unless K+ less than 3 mEq/L)

- Fatigue, malaise, muscle pain, weakness

Severe

- Progressive weakness, paresthesia, hypoventilation, arrhythmias, rhabdomyolysis

Signs and symptoms of hyperkalemia

- Weakness, flaccid paralysis of extremities, electrocardiogram (EKG) changes, paresthesias, confusion, shock, hypotension

Administration

- Administer all IV piggyback potassium chloride and maintenance fluids that contain potassium chloride with a concentration at or above 40 mEq/L to 60 mEq/L via an infusion pump.
- IV potassium chloride should always be diluted prior to administration. Potassium chloride should never be given IV push.
- Solutions containing potassium chloride should generally be administered at 10 mEq per hour. However, the following guidelines apply in some circumstances:
    - Administer via a peripheral line at a rate less than or equal to 10 mEq per hour.[5]
    - Administer via a central line at a rate less than or equal to 20 mEq per hour.[6]
    - 40 mEq/100 mL potassium chloride riders should always be administered via a central line because they are very concentrated and can cause vein irritation.

- Consider EKG monitoring if cardiac instability is a concern.
- The amount of potassium chloride added to solutions should not exceed
    - 60 mEq/L for maintenance fluids
    - 20 mEq/100 mL or 40 mEq/250 mL for administration through a peripheral line.[7]
    - 40 mEq/100 mL for administration through a central line.[8]
- Assess for multiple concomitant potassium chloride solutions (e.g., a 60 mEq potassium chloride rider is ordered for a patient currently receiving total parenteral nutrition containing 40 mEq potassium chloride).
- Do not crush or chew tablets.
- Give tablets with food or full glass of water to prevent gastrointestinal ulceration.

Monitoring

- Hyperkalemia can be asymptomatic and quickly develop into a fatal situation; therefore assess serum levels every four hours for patients receiving IV potassium supplementation (desired serum level is 3.5 mEq/L–5 mEq/L).
- Assess the IV site frequently for signs and symptoms of infiltration.
- It is difficult to correct hypokalemia in the presence of severe hypomagnesemia; therefore, monitoring and correcting magnesium levels is essential.[9]

Magnesium

Signs and symptoms of hypomagnesemia

- Hypokalemia and hypocalcemia
- Lethargy, confusion, ataxia, nystagmus
- Tremor, fasciculations, tetany, seizures
- Arrhythmias

Signs and symptoms of magnesium toxicity

- Hypotension
- Suppression of deep tendon reflexes
- Flushing, diaphoresis, hypothermia
- Cardiac, central nervous system, or respiratory depression

Administration

- Administer IV doses via an infusion pump.
- When administering magnesium intravenously, it is recommended to infuse at a rate no greater than 1 g per hour to prevent clinically significant hypotension and increased urinary losses of magnesium.
- For the treatment of preeclampsia, magnesium sulfate can be administered at a rate of up to 2 g per hour. A concentration of 25 g magnesium/250 mL NS is standard in many institutions. Only trained personnel should give it (via an infusion pump).
- 1 g–4 g mixed in 100 mL of Dextrose 5% in water or NS has been used to replace magnesium in patients with normal renal function; more conservative dosing is warranted in patients with renal dysfunction.
- Oral doses should be given with a full glass of water (8 oz) to prevent dehydration, as oral magnesium can cause diarrhea.
- IM administration must be into a large muscle mass, preferably into a gluteal site.
- Administration of oral magnesium salts with oral quinolone antibiotics or tetracyclines, such as levofloxacin or ciprofloxacin, may form nonabsorbable complexes resulting in decreased absorption of tetracyclines and quinolones. Do not administer oral magnesium salts within one to three hours of giving an oral tetracycline or oral quinolone.

Monitoring

- Keep in mind that replacement of magnesium may take three to seven days
- Monitor for symptoms of hypomagnesemia and magnesium toxicity

Phosphorus

Signs and symptoms of hypophosphatemia

- Progressive weakness, hypotension, hypoventilation, rhabdomyolysis, heart failure, paresthesia, dysarthria, confusion, stupor

Signs and symptoms of hyperphosphatemia

- Hypocalcemia, paresthesia, weakness, heaviness of legs, cardiac changes

Administration

- The oral powder pack formulations of phosphorus, such as Neutra Phos, must be mixed in a full glass (6 oz–8 oz) of water or skim milk prior to administration to ensure complete dilution.
- Oral phosphorus should be administered into at least three to four divided doses per day because they can be cathartic if too much is given in one dose.
- Only administer intravenously if patients are unable to tolerate oral doses.
- If IV therapy is necessary, sodium phosphate should be prescribed instead of potassium phosphate to avoid hyperkalemia.
- IV phosphate should always be dosed in mMol.
- Replace phosphate cautiously if the calcium level is elevated, because the relationship between calcium and phosphorus is not understood. Calcium phosphate may precipitate into the vasculature and result in organ injury.
- Administer IV phosphorus
    - via an IV infusion pump
    - at a maximum of 32 mMol per 24 hours to avoid toxicity
    - in 250 mL–500 mL of normal saline or dextrose 5% in water
    - over six to 12 hours (rapid infusion can cause phosphate toxicity)

Monitoring

- During IV administration, monitor plasma concentrations every six hours.[10]
- Because phosphorus preparations (both IV and oral) are only available in combination with sodium and/or potassium, these levels must also be monitored.
- Be aware that different forms and products do not always contain equal amounts of potassium and sodium and therefore are not interchangeable (e.g., K Phos Neutral contains 8 mMol phosphorus, 1.1 mEq potassium and 13 mEq sodium, while Neutra Phos packets contain 8 mMol phosphorus, 7 mEq of potassium, and 7 mEq of sodium).
- Monitor for signs and symptoms of hypophosphatemia and hyperphosphatemia. Note that symptoms are usually absent unless the phosphorus level is less than 1 mg/dL.[11]

Intravenous calcium

Signs and symptoms of hypocalcemia

- Hyperactive deep tendon reflexes, facial muscle spasm (Chvostek's sign), muscle and abdominal cramps, foot carpus spasm

Signs and symptoms of hypercalcemia

- Anorexia, confusion, constipation, drowsiness, hypertension, nausea/vomiting, premature ventricular contractions, polyuria

Administration

- Administer IV push calcium at a rate of 0.7 mEq/minute–1.8 mEq/minute (except in cardiac arrest). For example, one 10 mL vial of calcium gluconate 10% contains 4.65 mEq of calcium and should be administered over at least three minutes. If calcium is given too rapidly, sinus bradycardia or atrioventricular block, cardiac arrythmias, and/or cardiac arrest can occur, especially if the patient is also receiving digoxin.
- Call the physician or pharmacist for clarification if the desired salt is not specified when calcium is ordered. There is a three-fold difference in calcium between calcium gluconate and calcium chloride
- When given intravenously, local irritation can occur. IV injections should be given through a small needle into a large vein to avoid a rapid increase in local concentrations.
- Never administer intramuscularly or subcutaneously. Severe tissue necrosis and sloughing can occur.
- Replace calcium cautiously if the phosphorus level is elevated, because prescribers are unaware of interactions that occur between calcium and phosphorus. Calcium phosphate may precipitate into the vasculature and result in organ injury.

Monitoring

- Monitor for hypotension, dizziness, syncope, flushing, nausea, or vomiting. These symptoms can develop when administering calcium intravenously.
- Local irritation and necrosis can occur. Assess IV site frequently.

- Monitor renal function, as calcium levels can be affected by serum phosphorus and albumin levels. Specifically, calcium phosphate may precipitate in the vasculature, resulting in renal failure.[12]
- If your patient is also prescribed a calcium channel blocker, monitor blood pressure frequently as calcium supplementation antagonizes the effects of calcium channel blockers resulting in elevations in blood pressure.
- Use oral calcium supplements with caution in patients who have diarrhea; otherwise, malabsorption as fecal excretion can be increased.
- Monitor for signs and symptoms of hypocalcemia or hypercalcemia.

Sodium chloride 3% (hypertonic saline)

Signs and symptoms of hypernatremia

- Nausea, malaise, headache, lethargy, obtundation, seizures, coma, respiratory arrest

Administration

- Hypertonic solutions (sodium chloride greater than 0.9%) should only be used in initial treatment of acute, serious, and symptomatic hyponatremia. Therefore, hypertonic saline infusions are rarely necessary and should only be ordered by physicians experienced in the use of hypertonic saline.
- Administer only via a central line and infusion pump.
- Rate of infusion should not exceed 1 mEq/kg per hour.

Monitoring

- The symptoms that occur with hypernatremia are primarily neurologic and are related to both the severity and the rapidity of onset of the change in the plasma sodium concentration.
- Monitor serum sodium levels.
- A rare but dangerous side effect is osmotic demyelination syndrome. This syndrome is caused by an overly rapid increase in the plasma sodium concentration.

Exercise

For IV potassium chloride replacements containing potassium chloride 20 mEq in a 100 mL IV rider or 40 mEq potassium chloride in a 250 mL IV rider, how many mEqs can you infuse per hour via a peripheral line and a central line?

Answer provided on p. 57.

Summary points

- To ensure safe outcomes, take extra precautions when administering and monitoring electrolyte supplementation
- Always check the patient's most recent electrolyte level prior to administration and after treatment
- Clarify calcium orders that do not specify the salt (e.g., either calcium gluconate or calcium chloride) because they do not provide equal amounts of calcium
- If potassium is infused too rapidly or in excessive amounts, EKG changes and even cardiac arrest can result
- When administering electrolyte replacements intravenously, adhere to the maximum hourly dose limits
- Administer IV infusions of potassium, magnesium, phosphorus, and sodium chloride 3% (hypertonic saline) only via an infusion pump

References

1. M.R. Cohen and C.M. Kilo. "High-alert medications: Safeguarding against errors." In M.R. Cohen (Ed.), *Medication Errors.* Washington, DC: American Pharmaceutical Association, 1999.
2. Ibid.
3. Ibid.
4. Ibid.
5. M. Fotis, M.A. (Ed.) Optimizing medication use at NMH: Suggested guidelines for commonly encountered problems. Chicago: Northwestern Memorial Hospital, 2003.
6. Ibid.
7. Ibid.
8. Ibid.
9. Ibid.
10. Ibid.
11. Ibid.
12. See note 1 above.

Warfarin (Coumadin)

Why is warfarin identified as a high-alert medication?

Warfarin is an anticoagulant that exerts its action by interfering with the interconversion of vitamin K and vitamin K epoxide. Serious, even fatal, bleeding (if supratherapeutic) and thrombotic events (if subtherapeutic) can occur if it is prescribed, administered, or monitored inappropriately.

As you read this section, keep in mind the commonly reported problems associated with warfarin:

- Prescribers often fail to adjust doses properly in response to international normalization ratio (INR) results[1]
- Prescribers and other clinicians are not aware of the drugs and foods that may alter the anticoagulation effects of warfarin[2]
- There is confusion about which labs to order (e.g., activated Partial Thromboplastin Time is mistakenly ordered instead of an INR)
- INR levels are not monitored or evaluated properly[3]
- The clinician fails to acknowledge nonobvious signs and symptoms of bleeding
- The clinician fails to recognize that the influence of interactive drugs may take several days
- The clinician fails to consider that multiple inpatient hospital factors, such as a change to nothing by mouth (NPO), vomiting, and diarrhea, can affect hemostasis
- Tablets of different strengths are similar in color and may look alike

---

Case study I

A 65-year-old male is admitted to the hospital for a total hip replacement. He was started on warfarin postoperatively. On the third day after surgery, the dose was not given but was documented as administered. In response to his decreased INR value, the physician increased the dose because it seemed that the patient was resistant to the warfarin, even though the decreased INR level actually had been caused by a missed dose. The INR increased dramatically, putting the patient at high risk for hemorrhage.

Due to warfarin's narrow therapeutic range, its administration must be correctly documented.

Case study 2

A nurse on a surgical floor knows to give her patient a 5 mg dose of warfarin every night because he was admitted on that dose and has been taking it for years. She also notices that the INR on admit was therapeutic at 2.4. The patient has now been hospitalized for five days and is NPO with no further coagulation labs ordered. What should you do?

Remind the resident or managing physician that the patient's clinical status has changed since admission. Because he is NPO, his vitamin K stores are rapidly depleting, which affects the body's ability to make clotting factors. Recommend that the surgical team order an INR regularly because warfarin dose adjustments may be necessary.

Be aware that even if a patient is admitted with a stable warfarin regimen, the INR must continue to be monitored because multiple inpatient factors affect hemostasis. Examples of these factors include dietary changes and the addition of medications that may interact with warfarin.

Critical thinking

- Is the patient going for surgery or another procedure? If so, how long has the warfarin been on hold?
- Is the patient at increased risk for bleeding due to underlying conditions, food/medication interactions, or a change in dietary status?
- If a patient has been receiving warfarin as an outpatient, what time did he or she take the last dose?
- Are the appropriate labs ordered to effectively monitor a patient receiving warfarin?
- Is the patient on the same dose as he or she was at home? Is this appropriate?
- Prior to discharge, did the patient receive education about warfarin, including the risks of bleeding and the importance of monitoring, such as when and where to have the next INR drawn?
- Did you notify dietary services of vitamin K dietary restrictions?
- Did you verify whether other anticoagulants the patients may be receiving (e.g., heparin, low molecular weight heparin, oral agents, etc.) should be continued to avoid inadvertent concomitant anticoagulation?

Nursing implications

Administration

- Warfarin has a narrow therapeutic range and is long acting. Its anticoagulant effects can be affected by factors such as other medications, a change in dietary vitamin K (e.g., a change to NPO), and underlying disease processes.
- Administer warfarin at the same time every day; variable administration times can lead to false INR values.
- Document all administered doses. Even one extra dose can result in an elevated INR.
- Warfarin should be used with caution in conditions with blood loss or in which bleeding could put the patient at risk (e.g., surgery, peptic ulcer disease, and blood dyscrasias).
- In most cases, warfarin should be stopped four to five days prior to surgery. However, refer to clinician guidelines, as this decision depends on the patient's risk and INR.
- The elderly and those with congestive heart failure or liver disease are more susceptible to the effects of anticoagulants.
- Inform the patient of each day's INR and dose.
- More than 150 medications, including over-the-counter products and supplements, are reported to interact with warfarin.[4]

Drug interactions (common but not limited to)

Acetaminophen	Erythromycin/clarithromycin
Aspirin	Metronidazole
Sulfamethoxazole/trimethoprim	Nonsteroidal antiinflammatory drugs
Cimetidine	Levothyroxine
Ciprofloxacin/levofloxacin	Carbamazepine
Fluconazole	

Monitoring

- If a patient's dietary status changes, (e.g., change to NPO), the INR level should be checked regularly because changes in vitamin K stores affect the body's ability to make clotting factors.
- Assess INR values in relation to previous reported levels because the peak action of warfarin can take up to 72 hours or longer.
- The influence of other drugs on warfarin's mechanism of action may take several days. The INR should be repeated within a few days of initiating interacting medications.

- Communicate with the physician regarding concerns related to dose and appropriate monitoring.
- With every administered dose of warfarin, reinforce with the patient the risks of bleeding and the importance of compliance.
- Monitor for physical signs and symptoms of bleeding and document.

Signs and symptoms that may indicate bleeding that is not otherwise obvious:

Decreased blood pressure	Weakness
Dizziness	Shortness of breath
Decreased urine output	Headache
Decrease in hemoglobin and hematocrit	Pain in chest or abdomen
Mental status changes	

Obvious signs of bleeding:

Petechiae/excessive bruising	Dark, tarry stools
Coffee-ground emesis	Hematuria
Bleeding from gums	Nosebleed

Exercise

Upon admission, a 75-year-old patient states that she forgot to tell the admitting physician that she has been taking warfarin at home. She can't remember the dose but says the pill is round and "blueish" in color. What should you do? (More than one answer may be correct.)

    a. Assume that she is taking 4 mg at home because according to Clinical Pharmacology's Web site, the 4 mg warfarin tablet is blue, then call the physician to have it ordered.

    b. Consult a pharmacist to help determine the dose she has been taking at home and contact the physician to alert him or her to the situation.

    c. Have a family member bring in the most current medication bottle to verify the dose.

    d. Assume that the physician purposely did not order warfarin for this patient as she may be going for a procedure the next day.

Answer provided on p. 57.

Summary points

- Warfarin has a very narrow therapeutic range, so appropriately monitoring the INR level is critical.
- Because many factors initiated during hospitalization can alter warfarin's effects on hemostasis, such as drug interactions and dietary changes, continuous monitoring is vital.
- Frequently reinforce with the patient the risks of bleeding and the importance of compliance.

Exhibit 5.1

Potential interactions between dietary supplements and warfarin

Nutraceuticals, herbals, botanicals, traditional medicines, etc., are all considered dietary supplements under the Dietary Supplements Health and Education Act passed by the U.S. Congress in 1994. It is important to recognize that under this act, there is minimal regulation and lack of standardization of dietary supplement products. These are made by multiple manufacturers in a variety of preparations and strengths. Unlike prescription drugs, dietary supplements do not undergo FDA premarket review and approval based on evidence of safety and efficacy. Supplement quality is not validated by the FDA, and many quality problems have been well documented including lack of specified ingredients, excessive or inadequate amounts of specified ingredients, and various contaminants that might include active drugs. In addition, there are no legal requirements for supplement manufacturers to submit postmarketing reports to the FDA of adverse events, such as those caused by interactions with prescription drugs.

Below is a list of supplements that may interact with warfarin, altering warfarin's therapeutic effect. (List of supplements and interaction descriptions adapted from the Natural Medicines Comprehensive Database, *www.naturaldatabase.com*).
Please note the following:

- Supplement interactions with warfarin have been identified largely through published case reports rather than by systematic study of concurrent use. Nonetheless, if a supplement is on the list, it should be considered as having potential to disrupt warfarin therapy, which in the worst outcome, may result in either bleeding (from excessive warfarin effect) or thrombosis (from diminished warfarin effect).

- If a supplement is not on this list, one cannot, and should not, conclude that it means the supplement can be used safely together with warfarin.

- This is not an absolute, final list. No such list exists because new information is always becoming available. Therefore, it is important to recognize that this information is at best a snapshot taken at one point in time and that it is often necessary to check with up-to-date resources or consult with a health professional, such as a pharmacist, who has regular access to those resources. The Drug Information Center, of the Department of Pharmacy, can also help with such questions.

- It is important to recognize warfarin-supplement sequence variations and the implications of each (sequences 1 and 3 may cause the most serious adverse interaction outcomes):
    1. A patient already on a stable warfarin dose, now starts taking a supplement.
    2. A patient already on a supplement, now starts on warfarin.
    3. A patient already on both a stable warfarin dose and a supplement now stops taking the supplement.

- Decisions about starting, continuing, or stopping a particular supplement in a patient should be made with the managing physician, considering the most current information about the supplement (its quality and interaction and adverse effects profiles), and by taking a critical risk-benefit perspective. For example, if the benefits attributed to a supplement are not sufficiently supported by scientific evidence, then should the risk of concurrent use with warfarin be taken?

Exhibit 5.1	Potential interactions between dietary supplements and warfarin (cont.)
Supplement	**Interactions description**
Acerola	Concomitant use with acerola can reduce anticoagulant activity of warfarin due to acerola's vitamin C content.
Bishop's weed	Bishop's weed may have additive effects with anticoagulant or antiplatelet drugs and may increase the risk of bleeding. The bergapten constituent of bishop's weed has antiplatelet effects.
Boldo	Boldo may have additive effects with warfarin and may increase the INR.
Borage seed oil	Borage seed oil might prolong bleeding time and increase the risk of bruising and bleeding. It contains gamma linolenic acid, which can inhibit platelet aggregation.
Chlorella	Chlorella contains significant amounts of vitamin K, which may inhibit the anticoagulant activity of warfarin.
Cod liver oil	Concomitant use with anticoagulant or antiplatelet drugs can increase the risk of bleeding.
Coenzyme Q-10	Concomitant use can reduce the anticoagulation effects of warfarin. Coenzyme Q-10 is chemically similar to menaquinone and may have vitamin K–like procoagulant effects. Closely monitor patients taking warfarin and coenzyme Q-10. Dose adjustment may be necessary.
Danshen	Concomitant use increases the anticoagulant effects of warfarin and the risk of bleeding. There have been several case reports of increased INR after concomitant use of danshen and warfarin. Elevations in INR have occurred as early as three to five days after start of danshen. Danshen might also increase the rate of absorption and decrease the elimination rate of warfarin.
Devil's claw	Purpurea has occurred in a patient taking warfarin and devil's claw concurrently, suggesting over-anticoagulation.
Dong quai	Concomitant use increases the anticoagulant effects of warfarin and the risk of bleeding. Dong quai is thought to inhibit platelet activation and aggregation.
Fenugreek	Fenugreek might have additive effects with warfarin and increase the INR. Some fenugreek constituents have antiplatelet effects, although these might not be present in concentrations that are clinically significant. Fenugreek in combination with boldo has been associated with increased INR in a patient taking warfarin.
Flaxseed oil	There is some evidence that flaxseed oil can decrease platelet aggregation and increase bleeding time. Theoretically, using flaxseed oil in combination with anticoagulant or antiplatelet drugs might have additive effects and increase the risk of bleeding.
Garlic	Garlic can enhance the effects of warfarin as measured by the INR. Monitor patients using this combination closely. Dose adjustment may be necessary. Theoretically, garlic might also enhance the effects and adverse effects of other anticoagulant and antiplatelet drugs, including aspirin, clopidogrel (Plavix), enoxaparin (Lovenox), and others.
Ginger	Concomitant use of herbs that have coumarin constituents or affect platelet aggregation could theoretically increase the risk of bleeding in some people.
Ginkgo leaf (Ginkgo leaf extract)	Ginkgo leaf can increase the anticoagulant effects of warfarin and risk of bleeding.
Ginseng, panax	Concomitant use of ginseng and antiplatelet agents might increase the risk of bleeding.
Great plantain	Due to its vitamin K content, great plantain may antagonize drug effects when consumed in large amounts.
Green tea	Consumption of large amounts of green tea is reported to antagonize the effects of warfarin. This has been attributed to the vitamin K1 in green tea. However, as there is so little vitamin K1 in green tea, the interaction is more likely due to other constituents.
Kava	Preliminary evidence suggests that kava significantly inhibits cytochrome P450 enzymes, including CYP1A2, CYP2C9, CYP2C19, CYP2D6, and CYP3A4. Warfarin is metabolized CYP2C9.
Lycium	There is some evidence that lycium can increase the effects of warfarin and possibly increase the risk of bleeding. INR can increase in patients stabilized on warfarin who begin taking lycium. Researchers think that lycium inhibits cytochrome P450 (CYP) 2C9 (CYP2C9) metabolism of warfarin and increases warfarin levels.

	Potential interactions between dietary supplements and warfarin (cont.)

Exhibit 5.1

Supplement	Interactions description
Melatonin	There are isolated case reports of minor bleeding and decreased prothrombin activity in people taking melatonin with warfarin.
Milk thistle	There's preliminary evidence that milk thistle might inhibit the cytochrome P450 2C9 (CYP2C9) and cytochrome P450 3A4 (CYP3A4) enzyme.
Pantethine	Concomitant administration might increase the risk of bleeding. Some evidence suggests that pantethine reduces platelet aggregation. When taken concurrently with drugs that affect platelets or coagulation, it might have an additive effect.
Papaya	Concomitant use might potentiate the effects of warfarin, increasing the INR.
Rose hip	Concomitant use interacts with the vitamin C in rose hip. Large amounts of vitamin C can impair the warfarin response.
Saw palmetto	Theoretically, saw palmetto might increase the risk of bleeding when used concomitantly with these agents. Saw palmetto is reported to prolong bleeding time.
Smartweed	Concomitant use can decrease the anticoagulant effects of warfarin, possibly increasing the risk of clotting.
Soy	Soy milk has been reported to decrease the INR in a patient taking warfarin. The mechanism of this interaction is not known. Soy may also inhibit platelet aggregation.
St. John's wort	Concomitant use might decrease the therapeutic effects of warfarin. St. John's wort seems to significantly decrease INR. St. John's wort is thought to induce the cytochrome P450 (CYP) 2C9 (CYP2C9) enzyme, which is involved in warfarin metabolism. In addition, warfarin physically interacts with hypericin and pseudohypericin, active constituents of St. John's wort. When the dried extract is mixed with warfarin in an aqueous medium, up to 30% of warfarin is bound to particles, reducing its absorption. Taking warfarin at the same time as St. John's wort might reduce its bioavailability.
Stinging nettle (above ground parts)	There is some concern that stinging nettle might decrease the effects of anticoagulant drugs like warfarin. Stinging nettle contains a significant amount of vitamin K.
Turmeric	Concomitant use of turmeric might increase the risk of bleeding due to decreased platelet aggregation. Turmeric has been reported to have antiplatelet effects.
Vitamin A	Vitamin A toxicity is associated with hemorrhage and hypoprothrombinemia, possibly due to vitamin K antagonism. High doses of vitamin A (10,000 units/day for adults) could increase the risk of bleeding when taken with warfarin.
Vitamin C (Ascorbic Acid)	Concomitant use with large amounts of vitamin C might impair response to warfarin. Doses of vitamin C up to 10 g/day don't seem to affect coagulation time in patients taking warfarin. Higher doses of vitamin C might affect warfarin absorption or antagonize the anticoagulant effect of warfarin by an unknown mechanism.
Vitamin E	Use of more than 400 IU of vitamin E per day with warfarin might prolong prothrombin time, increase INR, and increase the risk of bleeding, due to interference with production of vitamin K–dependent clotting factors. The risk for vitamin E interaction with warfarin is greater in people who are already deficient in vitamin K.
Vitamin K	Vitamin K antagonizes the effects of oral anticoagulants like warfarin. Excessive vitamin K intake, either from supplements or from changes in diet, can reduce anticoagulation effect.
Wintergreen oil	Concomitant use of topical wintergreen oil-containing products and warfarin can increase INR and bleeding risk due to systemic absorption of the methyl salicylate contained in wintergreen oil. Topical analgesic gels, lotions, creams, ointments, liniments, and sprays can contain up to 55% methyl salicylate.

Source: List of supplements and interaction descriptions adapted from: Jellin JM, Gregory PJ, Batz F, Hitchens K, et al. Pharmacist's Letter/Prescriber's Letter Natural Medicines Comprehensive Database. Stockton, CA: Therapeutic Research Faculty, www.naturaldatabase.com, accessed 2004 January 20. Reprinted with permission from Bill Budris, RPh, Drug Information Center.

References

1. Clinical Pharmacology Database: Gold Standard Multimedia, Tampa, FL, 2004. Available online through NM Connect.
2. M. Leonard. "Interactions Between Herbs and Cardiac Medications." www.clevelandclinicmeded.com/medical_info/pharmacy/MarApr2001/herbs_cardiac.htm, accessed January 14, 2004
3. Natural Medicines Comprehensive Database. Stockton, CA: Therapeutic Research Faculty, 2004.
4. G.N. Scott and G.W. Elmer. Update on natural product—drug interactions." Am J Health Syst Pharm. 59 (2002): 339–47, www.ncbi.nlm.nih.gov/entrez/query.fcgi?cmd=Retrieve&db=PubMed&list_uids=11885397&dopt=Abstract

Neuromuscular blocking (paralytic) agents

Why are neuromuscular blocking agents identified as high-alert medications?

Neuromuscular blocking agents are used as an adjunct to general anesthesia during surgery or mechanical ventilation to provide skeletal muscle paralysis. Because they paralyze skeletal muscles, they are also used as an aid to tracheal intubation. Neuromuscular blocking agents have no intrinsic sedative effects: Thus, if administered alone, patients will be completely awake but unable to move. If prescribed, administered, or monitored inappropriately, respiratory arrest, muscle paralysis, and even death can occur.

Neuromuscular blocking agents:

Atracurium 10 mg/mL	Mivacurium 2 mg/mL
Doxacurium 10 mg/mL	Pancuronium 1 mg/mL, 2 mg/mL
Rocuronium 10 mg/mL	Cisatracurium 10 mg/mL, 2 mg/mL
Succinylcholine 20 mg/mL, 100 mg/mL	Vecuronium 10 mg/10 mL, 20 mg/10 mL

As you read this section, be aware of the commonly reported problems associated with neuromuscular blocking agents:

- Outside the operating room, neuromuscular blocking agents have been administered to patients who are not appropriately ventilated and therefore are at high risk for respiratory arrest[1]
- Extubation orders are acted upon prior to the discontinuation of a neuromuscular blocking agent
- Neuromuscular blockers have been confused with other medications, such as vaccines, leading to patient harm and even death[2]

Case study

A physician wanted to sedate a combative emergency room patient. A neuromuscular blocking agent was ordered and then subsequently administered by a nurse. The patient, who had not been intubated, coded, and suffered an anoxic insult.

Source: "Neuromuscular blocking agents—proposed labeling and packaging standards for medication error prevention." U.S. Pharmacopeia Quality Review (February 2000).

Critical thinking

- Is the patient ventilated properly prior to administering a neuromuscular blocking agent?
- Is the patient on any other medications that might enhance or prolong the neuromuscular activity of the agent?
- Is the patient also receiving appropriate sedation (i.e., opioid for pain/benzodiazepines for amnesia)? If not, he or she should be.
- Does the patient have underlying cardiovascular disease (heart rate and blood pressure changes may be of significance in these patients)?
- Is the neuromuscular blocking agent discontinued before mechanical ventilatory support is decreased or extubation is performed?

Nursing implications

Administration

- Only experienced clinicians familiar with the use of neuromuscular blocking agents should administer or supervise the use of these agents.
- Neuromuscular blocking agents should be administered only after proper sedative and pain medications have been instituted. Otherwise, the patient will be paralyzed but will feel pain to its fullest extent. Benzodiazepines are generally used to induce amnesia.
- Administer by rapid intravenous injection or by continuous intravenous infusion. Do not give intramuscular injections.
- Administer only if patient is properly ventilated.
- It is recommended that all neuromuscular blocking agents be labeled as such with a caution sticker (e.g., "Caution: Paralytic Agent").[3]

Exercise

True or false: Neuromuscular blocking agents should be automatically discontinued before the patient is extubated and removed from a ventilator.

Answer provided on p. 57.

Monitoring

- Adjust the rate of infusion according to patient response and clinical requirements.
- A peripheral nerve stimulator can be used to monitor the agent's effects.
- Check serum potassium concentrations prior to administration. Hypokalemia potentiates neuromuscular blockade with some neuromuscular blocking agents. Hyperkalemia and cardiac arrest can be induced with succinylcholine in patients who have had a stroke or spinal cord injury.
- Monitor heart rate, blood pressure, and mechanical ventilator status, as neuromuscular blocking agents increase the frequency of bradycardia and hypotension associated with opioids.

Summary points

- Many errors concerning the misuse of neuromuscular blocking agents, including accounts of serious injuries and fatalities, have been reported nationally.
- Proper ventilatory assistance and sedatives must be provided concurrently with neuromuscular blocking agents.
- As an extra method to alert the clinician, it is recommended that the pharmacy department label all paralytic infusions with a label stating, "Caution: Paralytic."
- Patients with cardiovascular disease or neurologic injury may experience severe hemodynamic instability after receiving neuromuscular blocking agents.

References

1. M.R. Cohen, and C.M. Kilo. "High-alert medications: Safeguarding against errors," *Medication Errors,* ed. M.R. Cohen, Washington, DC: American Pharmaceutical Association, 1999.
2. Ibid.
3. Ibid.

Chemotherapy agents

Why are chemotherapeutic agents identified as high-alert medications?

Chemotherapy is the use of cytotoxic or antineoplastic agents in the systemic or regional treatment of malignancy and other nononcologic indications. Due to the toxic nature of chemotherapy agents, if prescribed, administered, or monitored inappropriately, the results can be serious or even fatal.

As you read this section, be aware of the commonly reported problems associated with chemotherapeutic agents:

- Chemotherapy medications have a narrow therapeutic range. Therefore, these drugs carry a higher risk for causing harm or even death if used inappropriately.
- Chemotherapy regimens are typically complex, making them more prone to error.
- There may be confusion between the individual dose and the total dose over a course of therapy. (e.g., a woman died of a four-fold overdose of cyclophosphamide, which she was receiving to treat breast cancer. The error occurred because the total dose to be given over four days was given on each of the four days instead.[1])
- Many chemotherapy agents need to be dosed according to either body surface area (BSA) or body weight. Mix-ups can occur.
- Chemotherapy medications are often ordered by using brand names, nicknames, abbreviations, or acronyms (e.g., ESHAP) which can easily lead to misinterpretation and are not acceptable for prescribing.
- The doses are usually expressed in mg/m^2 or mg/kg. Confusion between these is common.[2]
- Vincristine has been inadvertently administered intrathecally, with fatal results.

Nursing implications

Case study

The perils of low-dose oral methotrexate are clearly evident in the dozens of fatalities reported in patients who have been prescribed methotrexate for alternative conditions.

For example, one patient died after he misunderstood the directions for use and took methotrexate

2.5 mg every 12 hours for six consecutive days, instead of 2.5 mg every 12 hours for three doses each week.

Another patient died after incorrectly reading the directions on a prescription bottle and taking 10 mg every "morning" instead of every "Monday." Errors also have been reported with hospitalized patients. In one case, the physician had properly recorded that the patient had been taking methotrexate 7.5 mg weekly as an outpatient. But when he prescribed three 2.5 mg tablets weekly, it was transcribed incorrectly as three times daily.

Source: "Look-alike/sound-alike drug names." Huntingdon Valley, PA: Institute for Safe Medication Practices, 2002 April 3.

This case study is an example of the how the complex nature of many chemotherapy regimens can make them more prone to error.

Critical thinking

- Are the chemotherapy orders written according to your institution's policy?
- Has the patient received this regimen before? If so, were there any complications?
- Was the correct measurement used to determine the dose (e.g., is it based on BSA, actual weight, or ideal weight)?
- When was the last regimen/cycle given? (including in outpatient settings, such as home or clinics)?
- Are the correct preparative/supportive medications ordered with the chemotherapy?
- Are labs current?
- What labs should continue to be monitored (e.g., are serum electrolyte levels being monitored appropriately)?

Administration

- According to the Oncology Nursing Society, only registered nurses who receive additional training, both didactic and clinical, can administer parenteral chemotherapy. Nonchemotherapy-validated registered nurses may administer oral or topical preparations.
- Do not crush oral tablets. Contact your pharmacy department, as they can prepare them under a biological safety cabinet.
- Chemotherapy should only be ordered using institution-established, standardized order templates or designated order sets in the computer. This will minimize the complexity of most chemotherapy regimens.
- No verbal orders or telephone orders should ever be accepted for chemotherapy except for discontinuing or holding orders. This will decrease misinterpretation. Verbal orders, however, may be taken to change supportive medications (e.g., change hydration fluids or add an antiemetic to the chemotherapy regimen).

- Verification of chemotherapy orders should require each nurse to
    - independently verify the original drug order (e.g., Is the order transcribed correctly? Is the attending physician's signature present?)
    - recalculate the BSA
    - recalculate the drug dose
    - verify that the dose on the drug label matches the original order
    - verify that three sets of pharmacy initials are present on the label
    - calculate the infusion pump rate
- All continuous infusions or intravenous piggyback agents should be administered via an infusion pump.
- The infusion pump rate should be independently checked prior to administration by two registered nurses as well as
    - with the original orders
    - when the bag is changed
    - at every shift change (incoming and off-going registered nurses), as needed.
- The most current lab values must accompany the order, either on the order or in the prescriber's note.
- All continuous infusion vesicant medications must be infused through a central venous access device that has a positive blood return. The blood return must be checked every two hours.
- It is recommended that all chemotherapeutic/cytotoxic drugs be sealed and packaged in a chemotherapy safe lock biohazard bag labeled as such.
- Chemotherapeutic/cytotoxic waste materials must be disposed of in a chemotherapy waste container. The waste container should never be stored in a patient's room.

Monitoring
- Assess the need to monitor electrolyte serum levels and fluid status.
- Monitor for signs of hypersensitivity/anaphylaxis (i.e., urticaria, localized/general itching, shortness of breath with or without wheezing, uneasiness/agitation, lightheadedness/dizziness, abdominal cramps, nausea, chills, symptoms of hypotension).[3]
- When your patient is receiving a vesicant, observe the site for infiltration/extravasation.
- Assess the patient's understanding of the treatment plan, expected outcomes, side-effect management, supportive medications, and potential risks. Provide education and written materials as indicated.
- Discharge education should include when to contact the physician and the contact phone number for follow-up or emergency use.

Exercise

The following order was just written for your patient:

VP-16 (50 mg/m²) 85 mg IV x 1 (day #1) BSA = 1.7 m²

What is wrong with this order?

Answer provided on p. 58.

Summary points

- Due to the narrow therapeutic range and extremely complex nature of most chemotherapy regimens, strict adherence to safe practices is essential when handling them.
- Verbal orders should only be accepted for holding or discontinuing chemotherapy orders.
- Infusion pump programming must always be independently checked by two registered nurses.
- Refer to chemotherapy drugs by their generic or chemical names. Brand names, abbreviations, and acronyms can lead to confusion.
- Educating your patients about their chemotherapy regimens, side effects, and discharge management procedures is crucial because knowledgeable patients can serve as the last line of defense in preventing an error.

References

1. M.R. Cohen, R.W. Anderson, R.M. Attilio, L. Green, R.J. Muller, and J.M. Pruemer. "Preventing medication errors in chemotherapy," *Medication Errors,* ed. M.R. Cohen. Washington, DC: American Pharmaceutical Association, 1999.
2. Ibid.
3. Oncology Nursing Society. *Cancer Chemotherapy Guidelines and Recommendations for Practice, 2nd ed.,* Pittsburgh, PA: Oncology Nursing Press, Inc., 1999.

Opioids

Contact the physician to get an order for a pain medication that does not contain acetaminophen. The patient has already received a total of 3650 mg of acetaminophen. Therefore, two more Norco would exceed the 4000 mg/day recommended limit for acetaminophen.

IV heparin

Administer the bolus, using a 5,000:1 concentration vial obtained from the pharmacy. Do not use the continuous infusion bag for boluses. The hourly rate equals 13mL/hour.

Insulin

False. Newer products such as Humalog, Lantus, and Novolog are clear but cannot be given intravenously.

Electrolytes

Peripheral line: administer at a rate less than or equal to 10 mEq/hour.

Central line: administer 40 mEq potassium chloride in a 100 mL IV rider at a rate less than or equal to 20 mEq/hour with electrocardiogram monitoring when appropriate.[1]

Warfarin (coumadin)

b. and c. Don't assume the dose is 4 mg because other tablets of warfarin are also "blueish" in color. The 6 mg warfarin tablet is blue-green and the 2.5 mg tablet is green. Consider that a blue-green or green tablet can be mistaken for the blue 4 mg tablet depending on the patient's eyesight, memory, and perception of color. This is a look-alike problem with warfarin tablets. Due to the narrow therapeutic range of warfarin, administering 6 mg instead of 4 mg can lead to an elevated international normalization ratio (INR). In addition, even though warfarin is often stopped prior to surgery or a procedure, this cannot always be assumed. Always contact the physician to confirm. Missing doses of warfarin can have severe consequences.

Neuromuscular blocking (paralytic) agents

True. Since the respiratory muscles are paralyzed, the patient can experience respiratory arrest.

Chemotherapy agents

Chemotherapy orders should never be written using abbreviations, acronyms, or nicknames. VP-16 is a common abbreviation for etoposide but should never be used when ordering or referring to it as this can easily lead to misinterpretation.

Reference

1. Fotis, M.A. (Ed.) *Optimizing medication use at NMH: Suggested guidelines for commonly encountered problems.* Chicago: Northwestern Memorial Hospital, 2003.

Nursing education instructional guide

Target audience:

- Directors of nursing
- Nurse managers
- Chief nursing officers
- Survey prep coordinators
- Vice presidents of nursing
- Directors of patient safety
- Directors of quality improvement

Training audience:

All nurses administering medications in the facility

Statement of need:

Medications labeled "high-alert" tend to have a higher risk of patient injury when involved in medication error. Patient safety is the underlying issue. Four of the Joint Commission on Accreditation of Healthcare Organizations' (JCAHO) seven National Patient Safety Goals cover medication administration. Medication safety has been on the front burner for years following the Institute of Medicine's (IOM) report, *To Err is Human*. The IOM report found that up to 98,000 deaths per year were the result of medical errors—making medical errors the 8th leading cause of death in the United States.

Educational objectives:

Upon completion of this activity, participants should be able to

- define the term "high-alert medication"

- describe the JCAHO's Patient Safety Goals related to medication administration

- identify commonly reported problems related to the use of opioids and describe why they are considered high-alert medications

- state specific safe practices that are recommended when administering and monitoring opioids

- identify commonly reported problems related to the use of intravenous heparin and describe why it is considered a high-alert medication

- state specific safe practices that are recommended when administering and monitoring intravenous heparin

- identify commonly reported problems related to the use of insulin and describe why it is considered a high-alert medication

- state specific safe practices that are recommended when administering and monitoring insulin

- identify commonly reported problems related to the use of electrolytes and describe why they are considered high-alert medications

- state specific safe practices that are recommended when administering and monitoring electrolytes

- identify commonly reported problems related to the use of warfarin and describe why it is considered a high-alert medication

- state specific safe practices that are recommended when administering and monitoring warfarin

- identify commonly reported problems related to the use of neuromuscular blocking agents and describe why they are considered high-alert medications

- state specific safe practices that are recommended when administering and monitoring neuromuscular blocking agents

- identify commonly reported problems related to the use of chemotherapy agents and describe why they are considered high-alert medications

- state specific safe practices that are recommended when administering and monitoring chemotherapy agents

Faculty:

Marla Husch, RPh
Jennifer M. Groszek, RN, BSN, MJ
Denise Rooney, RN, BSN, OCN

Accreditation/Designation statement:

This educational activity for 2.7 contact hour(s) is provided by HCPro, Inc. HCPro is accredited as a provider of continuing nursing education by the American Nurses Credentialing Center's Commission on Accreditation.

Disclosure statements:

Jennifer M. Groszek, Marla Husch, and Denise Rooney have signed forms declaring no commercial/financial vested interest in this activity.

Instructions for obtaining your nursing contact hours

To be eligible to receive your nursing contact hour(s) for this activity, you are required to complete the following:

1. Read the book
2. Complete the quiz
3. Complete the evaluation
4. Provide your contact information on the quiz and evaluation
5. Submit quiz and evaluation to HCPro, Inc.

Please provide all of the information requested above and mail or fax your completed quiz, program evaluation, and contact information to:

Robin L. Flynn
Manager, Continuing Education
HCPro, Inc.
200 Hoods Lane
P.O. Box 1168
Marblehead, MA 01945
Fax: 781/639-0179

If you have any questions, please contact Robin Flynn at 781/639-1872 or *rflynn@hcpro.com.*

Nursing education exam

Name: _____

Title: _____

Facility name: _____

Address: _____

Address: _____

City: _____ State: _____ ZIP: _____

Phone number: _____ Fax number: _____

E-mail: _____

Nursing license number: _____

(ANCC requires a unique identifier for each learner)

1. **A "high-alert medication" is one that**

   a. is frequently prescribed

   b. is frequently given in error

   c. has a high risk of causing harm when misused

   d. all of the above

2. **Errors involving high-alert medications have the same incident-reporting process as medication errors, near misses, and suspected adverse drug events.**

   a. True

   b. False

3. **The following safety principles are applicable with the administration of all medications:**

    a. Two unique identifiers, such as name and age, are assessed prior to medication administration

    b. The nurse receiving the telephone/verbal order performs a "read-back and verification" of the medication order

    c. The patient is informed of the drug, dose, potential side effects, and corresponding laboratory values, when appropriate

    d. All of the above

4. **An independent double check occurs when**

    a. a nurse checks that the pharmacy dispensed the correct medication

    b. one nurse reads to another nurse the amount of insulin he or she withdrew to verify that the correct dose will be administered

    c. two nurses separately calculate a dose without knowledge of each other's prior calculations

    d. a nurse places two check marks beside a documented administered dose to signify that he or she double-checked his or her own work

5. **After a change in a heparin dose, another activated Partial Thromboplastin Time (aPTT) should be drawn 12–24 hours later to evaluate the effect of the new dose.**

    a. True

    b. False

6. **Frequently, when transitioning from heparin to enoxaparin, a physician may prescribe both so that the two medication courses overlap.**

    a. True

    b. False

7. **When your patient is prescribed warfarin, which of the following safe practices apply?**

    a. Ensure that an aPTT is drawn on a consistent regimen

    b. Being cognizant that changes in diet can affect the international normalization ratio level

    c. Reinforce and educate the patient about the risk of bleeding and importance of compliance

    d. Answers b and c

    e. All of the above

8. Errors involving chemotherapy drugs

    a. can be catastrophic due to the drugs' narrow therapeutic range

    b. are often the result of the drugs' complex regimens

    c. are due to mix-ups between the appropriate routes of administration (e.g., inadvertent intrathe-cal administration)

    d. all of the above

9. **If your patient is receiving insulin as a scheduled medication, it is important to communicate regularly with the physician regarding any dietary intake changes.**

    a. True

    b. False

10. **A physician order indicates 40 milliequivalents (mEq) of potassium chloride intravenously because the patient has a serum potassium level of 3.3 mEq/L. He does not have a central line. Over what period of time should you administer the potassium chloride, and how often should the serum level be assessed?**

    a. Administer over two hours and check level every four hours

    b. Administer over four hours and check level every four hours

    c. Administer over four hours and check level every two hours

    d. None of the above

11. **A newly admitted patient has been taking MS Contin 30 milligrams (mg) two times a day. Now, he is taking nothing by mouth and needs to be converted to the intravenous (IV) route for pain control. An appropriate IV dose would be Morphine 30 mg IV twice a day.**

    a. True

    b. False

12. **Which of the following is not an acceptable patient identifier to be assessed prior to medication administration?**

    a. Medical-record number

    b. Age

    c. Room number

    d. Date of birth

Nursing education evaluation

Name: _____

Title: _____

Facility name: _____

Address: _____

Address: _____

City: _____ State: _____ ZIP: _____

Phone number: _____ Fax number: _____

E-mail: _____

Nursing license number: _____

(ANCC requires a unique identifier for each learner)

I. This activity met the following learning objectives:	Strongly disagree				Strongly agree
a. Define the term "high-alert medication"	1	2	3	4	5
b. describe the Joint Commission for the Accreditation of Healthcare Organizations' (JCAHO) Patient Safety Goals related to medication administration	1	2	3	4	5
c. identify commonly reported problems related to the use of opioids and describe why they are considered high-alert medications	1	2	3	4	5
d. state specific safe practices that are recommended when administering and monitoring opioids	1	2	3	4	5
e. identify commonly reported problems related to the use of intravenous (IV) heparin and describe why it is considered a high-alert medication	1	2	3	4	5

		Strongly disagree				Strongly agree
f.	state specific safe practices that are recommended when administering and monitoring IV heparin	1	2	3	4	5
g.	identify commonly reported problems related to the use of insulin and describe why it is considered a high-alert medication	1	2	3	4	5
h.	state specific safe practices that are recommended when administering and monitoring insulin	1	2	3	4	5
i.	identify commonly reported problems related to the use of electrolytes and describe why they are considered high-alert medications	1	2	3	4	5
j.	state specific safe practices that are recommended when administering and monitoring electrolytes	1	2	3	4	5
k.	identify commonly reported problems related to the use of warfarin and describe why it is considered a high-alert medication	1	2	3	4	5
l.	state specific safe practices that are recommended when administering and monitoring warfarin	1	2	3	4	5
m.	identify commonly reported problems related to the use of neuromuscular blocking agents and describe why they are considered high-alert medications	1	2	3	4	5
n.	state specific safe practices that are recommended when administering and monitoring neuromuscular blocking agents	1	2	3	4	5
o.	identify commonly reported problems related to the use of chemotherapy agents and describe why they are considered high-alert medications	1	2	3	4	5
p.	state specific safe practices that are recommended when administering and monitoring chemotherapy agents	1	2	3	4	5

		Strongly disagree				Strongly agree
2. Objectives were related to the overall purpose/goal of the activity		1	2	3	4	5
3. This activity was related to my nursing activity needs.		1	2	3	4	5
4. The exam for the activity was an accurate test of the knowledge gained.		1	2	3	4	5
5. The program avoided commercial bias or influence.		1	2	3	4	5
6. This program met my expectations.		1	2	3	4	5

7. **Will this learning activity enhance your professional nursing practice?**

   Yes   No

8. **How committed are you to making the behavioral changes suggested in this activity?**

   a. Very committed   b. Somewhat committed   c. Not committed

9. **This educational method was an appropriate delivery tool for the nursing/clinical audience.**

   Strongly disagree   1   2   3   4   5   Strongly agree

10. **Please provide us with your degree.**

    a. ADN   b. BSN   c. MSN   d. other

11. **Please provide us with your credentials.**

    a. LVN   b. LPN   c. RN   d. NP   e. other

12. **I found the process to obtain my continuing education credits for this activity easy to complete.**

   Strongly disagree   1   2   3   4   5   Strongly agree

13. **If you did not find the process easy to complete, which of the following areas did you find the most difficult?**

   a. Taking the exam

   b. Obtaining access to the online evaluation

   c. Completing the online evaluation

   d. Printing my certificate

   e. Understanding the instructions

14. **How much time did it take for you to complete this activity (this includes completing book, quiz, and evaluation)?**

   a. Less than 60 minutes

   b. 60–90 minutes

   c. 91–135 minutes

   d. 136–170 minutes

   e. more than 170 minutes

15. **Providing nursing contact hours influenced my decision to purchase this book.**

   Strongly disagree   1   2   3   4   5   Strongly agree

Notes